Craniosacral Therapy

The Complete Guide To Craniosacral Therapy Guide: Understanding The Tradition, Technique, And Transformative Healing

BANABAS WISDOM

Contents

Introductory

Craniosacral Therapy (CST) is an alternative therapeutic modality that centers on the manipulation of the cerebrospinal fluid and membranes comprising the craniosacral system, which safeguards the brain and spinal cord.

The therapeutic approach entails the application of non-invasive, gentle pressure to multiple anatomical regions, focusing specifically on the sacrum (a triangular bone located at the base of the vertebrae), head, and spine.

The following are fundamental tenets of Craniosacral Therapy:

• The craniosacral rhythm is a rhythmic pulsation believed to be generated by the cerebrospinal fluid in the central nervous system, according to practitioners. It is hypothesized that this rhythm serves as an indicator of nervous system health.

• The objective of the therapy is to augment the organic circulation of cerebrospinal fluid while also unclogging any impediments or obstructions within the craniosacral system. Practitioners identify and rectify imbalances through the use of soothing, hands-on techniques.

• Approach to Holistic Medicine: Craniosacral Therapy operates under the premise that the body operates in its entirety. In this modality, the therapist endeavors to attend to not only physical manifestations but also the fundamental psychological and emotional elements that might contribute to malafunction.

• The therapy promotes a state of relaxation and facilitates the discharge of tension, thereby stimulating the body's self-healing mechanisms.

Notably, there is ongoing debate regarding the efficacy and scientific foundation of Craniosacral Therapy. Although certain individuals have documented favorable experiences and advantages, the scientific community is generally skeptical of CST on account of the paucity of substantial empirical evidence substantiating its underlying principles and results.

It is imperative that, as with any alternative therapy, individuals exercise discernment and seek the advice of healthcare professionals before committing to any treatment options.

CHAPTER ONE
Applications, Scope, And Fundamentals

Fundamental tenets of Craniosacral Therapy:

1. Rhythmic Craniosacral Movement:

• The therapy is predicated on the notion that the motion of cerebrospinal fluid imparts a subtle, rhythmic pulsation to the craniosacral system. Using this rhythm as a diagnostic instrument, practitioners seek to restore the system's equilibrium.

2. Healing and innate health:

• CST functions on the premise that the human body possesses an intrinsic capacity for self-repair. Through the elimination of constraints within the craniosacral system, the therapeutic approach seeks to augment the intrinsic healing mechanisms of the body.

3. Holistic Methodology:

• The therapeutic approach considers the physical, emotional, and mental dimensions of the individual. By doing so, practitioners aim to treat symptoms of dysfunction rather than its underlying causes.

4. **Non-invasive, gentle techniques:**

• CST typically employs light palpation and manipulation of the head, spine, and sacrum in addition to the utmost delicacy of contact. The objective is to promote the alleviation of tension through non-coercive means.

The following describes the scope of craniofacial therapy:

1. Physical attributes:

• CST is occasionally employed to treat headaches, migraines, musculoskeletal discomfort, and temporomandibular joint (TMJ) disorders, among others.

2. Anxiety and Emotional Difficulties:

• The therapy endeavors to alleviate limitations encompassing the mental and emotional domains as well as the physical body. On occasion, it is utilized to mitigate the effects of emotional trauma, anxiety, and tension.

3. Neurological Pathologies:

• There is limited scientific evidence supporting the claims of some practitioners regarding the benefits of particular neurological conditions. In the context of CST, conditions such as concussions and specific developmental disorders have been mentioned.

4. Birth and Pregnancy Support:

• CST is occasionally applied to infants and expectant women for support. Practitioners assert that it can assist in alleviating pregnancy-related distress, facilitating childbirth, and treating infant ailments such as colic.

Strategies Employing Craniosacral Therapy:

1. Prevention and Wholeness:

• Certain individuals incorporate CST into their wellness regimen with the intention of averting health complications and enhancing general wellness.

2. Complementary treatment consists of:

• Complementary therapy (CST) is frequently regarded as an adjunct to conventional medical procedures. It is critical for individuals to engage in dialogue with healthcare professionals and incorporate CST into a comprehensive healthcare plan when deemed appropriate.

3. Stress Mitigation:

• Certain individuals hold the belief that the mild characteristics of CST facilitate tension reduction and relaxation, thereby augmenting one's general state of well-being.

• Although certain individuals have reported favorable experiences with Craniosacral Therapy, the body of scientific evidence substantiating its effectiveness is relatively scant. The therapy's lack of ubiquitous acceptance in the medical community necessitates a critical approach from individuals, who should evaluate it in conjunction with conventional medical care. It is imperative to seek guidance from healthcare professionals prior to undertaking any alternative or complementary therapies.

Anatomy Of The System Craniosacral

The craniosacral system is a physiological configuration of the human body comprising primarily structures related to the central nervous system and the fluid-filled cavities that provide protection and encirclement to it. Critical elements comprising the craniosacral system comprise:

1. The Cranial Bones:

• Comprised of multiple bones, the cranium, also known as the skull, serves to enclose and safeguard the brain. The frontal bone, parietal bones, temporal bones, occipital bone, sphenoid bone, and ethmoid bone comprise these bones.

2. CSF: Cerebrospinal fluid

• It's an aqueous, transparent substance that envelops the brain and spinal cord. It safeguards and imparts buoyancy to the central nervous system. Cerebrospinal fluid (CSF) is generated in the ventricles of the brain and is transported via the subarachnoid space around the brain and spinal cord.

3. The Dura Mater:

• The dura mater is the most durable and outermost of the three meningeal layers, which are the membranes encompassing the spinal cord and brain. An enveloping barrier is formed around the brain and spinal cord.

4. The Arachnoid Mater:

• The arachnoid mater comprises the meninges' intermediate layer. Its location intermediate to the pia mater and dura mater. Subarachnoid space is the region encompassing cerebrospinal fluid that is situated between the arachnoid mater and the pia mater.

5. The Pia Mater:

• As the innermost layer of the meninges, the pia mater adheres directly to the brain and spinal cord surfaces. Vascular and delicate in nature.

6. The Craniosacral System comprises the following elements:

• Owing to the connection between the cranium (skull) and the sacrum (the triangular bone situated at the base of the vertebrae), the term "craniosacral" is derived.

The dura mater is a continuous sheath that extends from the cranium to the sacrum. The pulsatile cadence of the cerebrospinal fluid within this system is referred to as the craniosacral rhythm.

7. Rhythmic Craniosacral Movement:

• The craniosacral rhythm refers to the delicate and rhythmic pulsation that arises from the cerebrospinal fluid production and circulation within the craniosacral system. This rhythm is employed by Craniosacral Therapy practitioners for diagnostic and therapeutic purposes.

A comprehensive comprehension of the anatomical components and rhythms that comprise the craniosacral system is imperative for practitioners of Craniosacral Therapy, given the intricate nature of the work involved. It is imperative to acknowledge that although the anatomical aspects of Craniosacral Therapy are firmly established, the therapeutic assertions linked to this modality are a matter of contention among the medical and scientific communities.

CHAPTER TWO
Rhythmic Craniosacral

The craniosacral rhythm is an imperceptible, pulsating sound that is hypothesized to originate from the cerebrospinal fluid (CSF) motion within the craniosacral system.

Craniosacral Therapy (CST), an alternative therapeutic approach that seeks to identify and manipulate this cadence in order to enhance overall health and wellness, places significant emphasis on this rhythm.

Key elements regarding the craniosacral rhythm are as follows:

1. Circulation and Origination:

• The craniosacral rhythm is implicated in cerebrospinal fluid production, absorption, circulation, and absorption.

Cerebrospinal fluid is generated within the ventricles of the brain and subsequently reabsorbed into the circulation after circulating throughout the brain and spinal cord within the subarachnoid space.

2. Synchronous Pulse:

• According to proponents of CST, the craniosacral rhythm is a cyclical, imperceptible pulsation that can be palpated. It is asserted that this pulsation is unique in comparison to other physiological frequencies, including respiration and heart rate.

3. Instrument of Diagnostic and Therapeutic Value:

• The craniosacral rhythm is a diagnostic instrument utilized in Craniosacral Therapy to evaluate the mobility and health of the craniosacral system. Practitioners employ their hands to palpate and perceive the rhythm with care, with the intention of identifying any irregularities or limitations.

4. Releasing and Equilibrating Tension:

• Through the release of restrictions and restoration of equilibrium to the craniosacral system, CST aims to improve the cadence of the craniosacral system. In order to improve the passage of cerebrospinal fluid, practitioners manipulate the tissues and structures associated with the craniosacral system using gentle, manual techniques.

5. Compatibility with the Nervous System:

• Advocates of CST posit that there exists a correlation between the operation of the central nervous system and the craniosacral rhythm. They hold the belief that by manipulating this cadence, one can potentially effectuate a beneficial transformation on the nervous system's overall health and functionality.

6. Stewardship and Controversy:

• In the scientific and medical communities, the existence of the craniosacral rhythm and the effectiveness of craniosacral therapy are contentious and sceptical topics. Critics contend that the objective measurement of the craniosacral rhythm is hampered by its subtlety, and that practitioners' purported therapeutic benefits are not substantiated by substantial scientific evidence.

Individuals contemplating Craniosacral Therapy should adopt a discerning perspective, taking into account both the testimonies of practitioners and the scientific evidence substantiating its tenets and results.

It is recommended to seek guidance from healthcare professionals and evaluate complementary approaches as part of a comprehensive healthcare regimen, prior to implementing any alternative therapy.

Fundamental Craniosacral Therapy Techniques

Craniosacral Therapy (CST) encompasses a series of non-invasive, manual techniques designed to evaluate and modify the frequencies associated with the craniosacral system.

Although practitioners may employ distinct techniques, the following are fundamental techniques that are frequently utilized in Craniosacral Therapy:

1. Soft Touch:

- Practitioners employ an exceptionally light contact, frequently characterizing their technique as considerably more gentle than a conventional massage. Without exerting force, this contact is intended to activate the body's self-correction mechanisms.

2. Attention:

• In order to "listen" to the craniosacral rhythm, practitioners place their hands gingerly on particular body parts, including the sacrum, head, and spine. Palpating for subtle movements and alterations in the craniosacral rhythm constitutes this method of listening.

3. Cranial traction:

• The therapist may employ mild pressure or contact on the cranium (skull) in order to perceive and manipulate the cranial bones' motion. The purpose of these holds is to promote the alleviation of stress and constraints.

4. Utilizing Sweeping Motions:

• Professionals may employ expansive hand gestures in order to replicate the organic motions of the craniosacral rhythm. Tracing the contours of the skull or vertebrae with light, rhythmic movements may be required.

5. Facial Disclosures:

• Fascia, an interconnecting tissue, provides support and envelops a multitude of anatomical components. Craniosacral Therapy (CST) may encompass non-invasive techniques aimed at mobilizing the fascia by alleviating constriction.

6. Balancing Methods:

• In order to achieve equilibrium in the craniosacral system, the therapist may employ techniques that target areas of restriction or asymmetry. This may entail coordinating the activity of various body segments in order to attain a state of balance.

7. Energy Capacity:

• Certain practitioners integrate the notion of subtle energy into their practice by employing light holds as a means to counterbalance and augment the energy circulation within the organism.

8.   SOT: Sacro-Occipital Technique

- An instance of CST that emphasizes the correlation between the sacrum (the anatomical base of the vertebrae) and the occiput (the posterior portion of the skull) is this particular technique. SOT consists of delicate adjustments utilized to rectify spinal and pelvic imbalances.

9. Tube Dural Rocking:

- This methodology incorporates nuanced motions with the objective of impacting the dura mater, which is the outermost layer of the meninges, as well as the cerebrospinal fluid flow.

10. Thymus Rotation:

• Certain practitioners integrate methods to subtly stimulate the thymus gland, a gland that some consider to possess immune-modulating properties.

Notably, within the scientific and medical communities, the efficacy of these techniques and the underlying principles of Craniosacral Therapy are subjects of contention. Those who are intrigued by CST ought to adopt a receptive mindset and contemplate seeking guidance from healthcare experts to ascertain its appropriateness in conjunction with their comprehensive healthcare regimen.

CHAPTER THREE
Assessment And Analyses

Practitioners of Craniosacral Therapy (CST) customarily perform assessments and evaluations in order to gain insight into the client's state of being, pinpoint regions of tension or restriction, and formulate an intervention strategy.

CST evaluations frequently incorporate a blend of palpation, listening to the craniosacral rhythm, and observation. The assessment and evaluation procedure in Craniosacral Therapy consists of the following critical elements.

1. History of Health and Intake:

• The initial step involves the practitioner collecting pertinent details regarding the client's general well-being, medical background, and any particular ailments or symptoms that may be present. This may encompass details pertaining to previous medical procedures, surgical interventions, and present medication regimens.

2. Client Consultation:

• Owing to a comprehensive dialogue with the client, the practitioner is better able to discern their apprehensions, symptoms, and objectives for the session. This may entail inquiring about pain, tension, emotional health, and any other pertinent variables.

3. An observation is made:

• As part of the assessment, the practitioner monitors the client's body alignment, movement patterns, and posture. Visual evaluation has the capacity to unveil potential sources of tension or imbalance.

4. As one observes the Craniosacral Rhythm:

• CST is distinguished by the capacity of the practitioner to palpate and listen to the craniosacral rhythm. This procedure entails lightly touching designated anatomical regions, including the cranium, spine, and sacrum, with the intention of perceiving subtle vibrations and patterns linked to cerebrospinal fluid.

5. Upon palpation:

• Practitioners palpate various body parts, including the cranium, spine, and limbs, with a light touch. Their objective is to detect regions of tension, restriction, or asymmetry via palpation.

6. Mobility Evaluation:

• An essential element entails evaluating the mobility of cranial bones, sacrum, and additional structures. The practitioner may assess the quality and range of motion in various body parts through the use of light movements.

7. Facial Evaluation:

• The fascial system may be evaluated by the therapist in order to identify any areas of fascial restriction or tension. Connective tissue that envelops and provides support for organs, tendons, and other structures is known as fascia.

8. Emotional and Sensory Awareness:

• Certain practitioners direct their focus towards the sensory and emotional experiences of the client throughout the session. This may entail inquiring about bodily sensations, emotional states, or mental fluctuations.

9. Setting Collaborative Objectives:

• The treatment objectives are established in collaboration between the practitioner and client, in light of the assessment findings. This may encompass the management of particular symptoms, enhancement of general health, or facilitation of relaxation.

10. Evaluation Reassessment:

• The practitioner may reevaluate the client's response to the treatment and modify their approach as necessary during the session. Facilitating the body's self-correction mechanisms is the objective.

Despite the fact that a considerable number of clients attest to the benefits of Craniosacral Therapy, the scientific literature is scant in support of its effectiveness.

Individuals who are contemplating CST should engage in candid communication with their practitioners, consult with healthcare professionals, and gather information from reputable sources in order to make well-informed decisions regarding their healthcare.

Ailments And Conditions Treated With Craniosacral Therapy

Craniosacral Therapy (CST) is frequently advocated as a comprehensive method of wellness that has the potential to alleviate numerous conditions and enhance general health.

Nevertheless, it is imperative to acknowledge that the scientific literature pertaining to the efficacy of CST for particular ailments is scant, and personal encounters with the treatment may differ. The following conditions and maladies are mentioned by proponents of Craniosacral Therapy as potential targets:

1. Migraines and Headaches:

• Certain people opt for CST as a means of mitigating tension headaches and migraines. By releasing tension in the craniosacral system, practitioners may be able to alleviate headache symptoms.

2. Persistent Pain:

• As an additional method of managing chronic pain conditions such as back pain, cervical pain, and joint pain, CST is occasionally implemented. The objective of therapy is to facilitate relaxation and alleviate inhibitions.

3. Disorders of the Temporomandibular Joint (TMJ):

• Craniosacral Therapy is a treatment option that may be contemplated by those who are afflicted with mandible pain, clicking, or discomfort that is commonly associated with temporomandibular joint disorders. The objective of these techniques is to alleviate tension in the mandible and its environs.

4. Anxiety and Stress:

• Advocates contend that the tranquility and gentle pressure fostered by CST could potentially mitigate symptoms of tension and anxiety. The objective of the treatment is to alleviate both physical and emotional strain.

5. Sleep disturbances:

• Certain people opt for CST in order to resolve sleep-related concerns, including insomnia or challenges with initiating sleep. The purpose of treatment is to induce nervous system equilibrium and relaxation.

6. Psychopathic Trauma:

• Practitioners of CST frequently highlight the holistic aspect of the treatment, hypothesizing that it might assist people in releasing bodily-held emotional trauma and tension.

7. PTSD: Post-Traumatic Stress Disorder

• CST may be beneficial for individuals with PTSD, according to some proponents, because it addresses both the physical and emotional aspects of trauma. However, there is limited scientific evidence to corroborate this claim.

8. Concerning Infants and Pediatrics:

• CST is occasionally applied to children and infants to treat conditions including colic, difficulty suckling, and developmental issues. Professionals may employ delicate techniques in order to promote the child's overall welfare.

9. Injuries to the Head and Concussions:

• Certain individuals opt for CST as a therapeutic intervention following head injuries or concussions, anticipating that it might facilitate tension relief and promote the recovery process. It is critical to emphasize that head injuries require immediate medical attention and evaluation.

10. Overall Health and Preventive Measures:

• Certain individuals utilize Craniosacral Therapy as a broad-ranging wellness regimen, with the objective of preserving bodily equilibrium and averting potential health complications.

It is critical to approach Craniosacral Therapy with the knowledge that there is no solid scientific consensus regarding its efficacy. Although certain individuals attest to positive experiences and advantages, others might not perceive it as efficacious.

Those who are contemplating CST should seek the advice of healthcare professionals, maintain open lines of communication with practitioners, and, when applicable, incorporate the therapy into their comprehensive healthcare regimen.

CHAPTER FOUR
Craniosacral Therapy Integrated With Additional Modalities

The integration of Craniosacral Therapy (CST) with other conventional or complementary modalities is a prevalent strategy within the realm of holistic healthcare.

Numerous individuals elect to integrate CST with additional therapeutic modalities or medical interventions in order to tackle an array of physical and emotional concerns. The following factors should be taken into account when contemplating the integration of

Craniosacral Therapy with other modalities:

1. Interactions with Healthcare Professionals:

• It is imperative that individuals undergoing conventional medical treatment or therapy for a particular ailment maintain open lines of communication with their healthcare providers.

Disseminate your enthusiasm regarding Craniosacral Therapy and engage in a dialogue regarding its potential to augment or harmonize with your current therapeutic regimen.

2. Care Collaboration:

• Working with a team of healthcare providers, each of whom contributes their own area of expertise to address a distinct aspect of your health, constitutes collaborative care.

Professionals in the fields of medicine, physical therapy, massage therapy, and mental health may be included. One element that can be incorporated into this collaborative approach is CST.

3. Physical Treatment:

• It is common practice to combine Craniosacral Therapy and physical therapy, particularly when addressing musculoskeletal conditions. CST practitioners and physical therapists may collaborate to treat mobility, alignment, and pain concerns.

4. Care by Chiropractic:

• Certain individuals opt to integrate Craniosacral Therapy with chiropractic treatment. Both modalities are centered around the musculoskeletal system; therefore, their integration could potentially target concerns associated with nervous system functionality and spinal alignment.

5. Using massage therapy:

• CST and massage therapy both aim to induce relaxation and alleviate tension. By incorporating both modalities, a holistic strategy for addressing muscular and fascial issues may be achieved.

6. The acupuncture modality:

• The combination of CST and acupuncture is an additional method. By integrating CST with acupuncture, which concentrates on the flow of energy (qi) in the body, a holistic approach to promoting balance may be achieved.

7. The provision of mental health counseling:

• A beneficial approach is to integrate Craniosacral Therapy with mental health counseling or psychotherapy when addressing concerns associated with stress, anxiety, or trauma. This methodology encompasses the psychological and physiological dimensions of wellness.

8. Mind-Body and Yoga Practices:

• By engaging in mind-body disciplines such as yoga, meditation, and CST, one can optimize their overall well-being through the integration of physical, emotional, and spiritual dimensions.

9. Provision of Nutritional Support:

• It is advisable to integrate nutritional counseling or dietary modifications in conjunction with CST in order to achieve a holistic approach to health and well-being.

10. Holistic Methods of Wellness:

• Incorporating lifestyle adjustments, including the adoption of a nutritious diet, consistent participation in physical activity, and adequate rest, can enhance the efficacy of Craniosacral Therapy and promote holistic health.

When considering the integration of modalities, it is critical to adopt an open and well-informed perspective. Communicate your objectives and personal preferences to each practitioner, and ensure that all members of your healthcare team are operating under the same page.

Coordination is required when integrating modalities to guarantee that the various approaches contribute synergistically to your overall health and wellness objectives.

Craniosacral Therapy Throughout An Individual's Life

Craniosacral Therapy (CST) is a comprehensive framework that is frequently applied to individuals of all ages, ranging from neonates to the elderly.

In spite of the fact that the precise methodologies and objectives may differ contingent upon the age and unique requirements of each practitioner, the overarching aim of CST is to rectify physical, emotional, and energetic imbalances that exist within the craniosacral system.

The application of CST can be observed in various life stages as follows:

Minors and Infants:

1. Infant Trauma:

• Occasionally, CST is employed to treat the consequences of birth trauma on neonates. Relaxation and support for the craniosacral system of the neonate are achieved through the use of gentle techniques.

2. Issues with the Digestive System and Colic:

• Parents may opt for CST as a means to treat infant complications such as colic or digestive issues. Practitioners employ delicate techniques to facilitate the infant's systemic equilibrium and relaxation.

3. Challenges of Breastfeeding:

• CST might be a viable option to consider for infants who are encountering challenges with the act of lactation. The objective of the treatment is to alleviate tension or constriction in the cranium, jaw, and mouth.

4. Delays in development include:

• Some parents consider CST for children with developmental delays as a supplementary method. The objective of practitioners is to promote holistic health and mitigate any potential physical limitations.

5. Infections of the Ear and Respiratory Problems:

• CST is occasionally employed in conjunction with medical interventions to treat conditions such as respiratory issues or ear infections. The objective of the treatment is to induce balance and relaxation in the head and neck.

Adolescents and Children:

1.   Individuals with learning disabilities:

• Parental involvement in CST for children with cognitive disabilities may promote the children's general health. Therapy is frequently administered in a holistic fashion, encompassing both physical and emotional dimensions.

2. Stress and Anxiety:

• Children and adolescents who are experiencing anxiety or tension may benefit from CST. The delicate techniques are designed to facilitate nervous system equilibrium and relaxation.

3. Sports and Injuries:

• CST may be a viable option for adolescents and children engaged in athletic activities in order to mitigate injuries, facilitate recuperation, and augment general physical health.

4. Overall Emotional Health:

• CST is occasionally employed as a means to promote the emotional welfare of infants and adolescents. Emotional tension may be addressed through the utilization of subtle craniosacral system components by practitioners.

Adults (adult):

1. Persistent Pain:

• Chronic pain patients in adulthood may benefit from investigating CST as a supplementary modality. The objective of practitioners is to facilitate relaxation and alleviate tension within the craniosacral system.

2. Anxiety and Stress:

• Adult individuals who are grappling with tension and anxiety frequently seek CST. The therapy potentially provides a holistic and compassionate method for addressing these concerns.

3. Migraines and Headaches:

• CST may be a viable option for individuals suffering from headaches or migraines as it alleviates tension in the head and neck and enhances general health.

4. Following a traumatic event:

• CST is occasionally investigated in the context of a comprehensive strategy for managing post-traumatic stress. The objective of the therapy is to facilitate the discharge of accumulated stress and trauma.

The elderly:

1. Concerns Regarding Arthritis and Joints:

• CST might be a viable option for the elderly demographic in order to mitigate concerns associated with arthritis and joint discomfort. The goal of the moderate techniques is to facilitate relaxation and mobility.

2. Mobility and equilibrium:

• Seniors who are grappling with challenges related to balancing and mobility may benefit from CST as a means to promote holistic physical health and alleviate constraints in the craniosacral system.

3. Chronic Illnesses:

• As a supplementary method, CST is occasionally pursued by patients who suffer from chronic health conditions. The goal of practitioners is to promote well-being and quality of life in general.

4. Emotional Assistance:

• CST may provide elderly individuals with emotional support by attending to the emotional dimensions of the aging process and encouraging a state of tranquility and equilibrium.

Although a considerable number of individuals attest to the benefits of Craniosacral Therapy, the scientific community has provided scant support for its effectiveness in treating particular conditions.

When contemplating CST, individuals ought to seek guidance from healthcare professionals, maintain open lines of communication with practitioners, and regard the therapy as a singular element of a comprehensive healthcare regimen.

Summary

A holistic approach, Craniosacral Therapy (CST) seeks to rectify energetic, physical, and emotional imbalances within the craniosacral system.

Although the therapy is administered to individuals of all ages, including neonates and the elderly, its efficacy and underlying principles continue to generate controversy in the scientific and medical communities.

Advocates of CST contend that it potentially provides advantages including alleviation of pain, mitigation of tension, and promotion of emotional welfare. The therapeutic approach's mild methodologies, centred around the release of tension and the craniosacral rhythm, resonate with individuals in search of non-intrusive and holistic methods to well-being.

Craniosacral therapy must be approached, nevertheless, with a critical and well-informed mindset. Limited scientific evidence supports its efficacy for particular conditions, and individual responses to the treatment may differ. It is advisable to incorporate CST into conjunction with other modalities and maintain transparent communication with healthcare providers in order to adopt a holistic and cooperative approach to health and wellness.

Similar to any healthcare procedure, prioritizing one's individual requirements, seeking guidance from healthcare experts, and exercising sound judgment are essential when contemplating the integration of Craniosacral Therapy into a comprehensive wellness regimen.

Ongoing research in the field of alternative and complementary therapies may yield additional insights into the mechanisms and efficacy of Craniosacral Therapy in the coming years.

THE END